SEEING THE WORLD DIFFERENTLY

Inside the Beautiful Mind of a Child with Autism

JIL LASACA, OTR

MARIA SHINE MANHILOT, OTR

ISBN: 978-1-967348-00-8 (Paperback)
ISBN: 978-1-967348-01-5 (e-Book)

Any references to historical events, real people, or real places are used fictitiously. Names, characters, and places are products of the author's imagination.

Printed by Iconic Global Media, Inc., in the United States of America

Iconic Global Media, Inc.
201 N. Brand Blvd., Suite 200,
Glendale, California 91203 USA
+1 (818) 459-5008
www.iconicglobalmedia.com

About The Authors

Jil Lasaca is an Occupational Therapist and co-founder of Bluebonnet Caring Home (assisted living facility) in Texas. She is the former Editor in Chief of Asian Beat Magazine. She is a real estate investor and a book lover.

Maria Shine Manhilot is a licensed Occupational Therapist in California. She has more than two decades of experience in the field. She loves cooking homemade recipes.

INTRODUCTION

Children with autism are a gift to the world, bringing with them unique perspectives, talents, and stories. Some are delightfully funny and quirky; others are deeply creative and artistic. Many have minds brimming with extraordinary ideas. Yet, they also face significant challenges.

Navigating social situations and emotional expressions can be difficult for them. They may struggle to interpret non-verbal cues or understand and respond to the emotions of others. Patterns of repetitive behavior and restricted interests are common, as are difficulties initiating and maintaining friendships. Many are hypersensitive to their surroundings— everyday sensations like sounds, bright lights, tastes, and textures can feel overwhelming. In their world, everything appears magnified, more intense, and sometimes harder to process.

Raising a child with autism is a journey like no other. It's filled with challenges but also immense growth and transformation. Caring for an autistic child reshapes a parent's perspective on life, teaching them profound patience, persistence, and a capacity for compassion and forgiveness they never thought possible.

However, this journey can also be confusing and exhausting. It requires endless energy and time. Parents and caregivers often ride a rollercoaster of emotions, experiencing guilt, anxiety, sadness, and frustration alongside joy and discovery.

What compelled us to write this book?

We took this journey of writing for personal and professional reasons. Jil Lasaca's early work as a newly minted Occupational Therapist at Northern Mindanao Medical Center, brought her unique world of discovery and growth while working with children with special needs at the clinic. Maria Shine's reason is deeply personal as she has a niece who was diagnosed with the spectrum.

As Occupational Therapists, we bring a unique holistic, child-centered approach to our work, focusing not just on the child's challenges but also on their strengths. On most occasions, we work with allied professionals including physical and speech therapists, early intervention specialists, and developmental specialists to address various areas of function for every child.

Occupational therapists (OTs) play a vital role in supporting children with autism spectrum disorder (ASD). Their work focuses on helping children develop the skills they need to navigate daily life, enhance their independence, and improve their overall quality of life. OTs use evidence-based approaches to address the unique challenges and strengths of each child, tailoring interventions to meet their individual needs. By fostering independence, improving functional skills, and enhancing participation in meaningful activities, OTs make a significant difference in the lives of children with autism and their families.

As we worked with children with autism, we witnessed firsthand the profound impact that early intervention, compassion, and understanding can have on their lives. Their unique perspectives, strengths, and challenges inspired us to share our knowledge and experience with others, hoping to make a difference in the lives of these incredible individuals.

The resilience, adaptability, and determination of children with autism and their families left an indelible mark in our hearts, motivating us to write a book that would honor their journeys and provide support to those who need it most.

Who is the book for?

Through our book, we aim to empower parents, caregivers, and professionals with the tools, strategies, and insight needed to create a more inclusive, accepting, and supportive environment for children with autism to thrive.

By sharing our unique life experiences as therapists and the stories of these remarkable children and their families, we hope to inspire a deeper understanding, appreciation, and celebration of neurodiversity, promoting a world where every individual can reach their full potential.

We wrote this book to support parents and caregivers of children with autism, offering them guidance and comfort. It is for educators, therapists, and advocates who aspire to create learning environments for these children to function in areas of self-care and community integration. It is also for anyone seeking to better understand the inner world of an autistic child—because their minds hold incredible depth and beauty, waiting to be appreciated.

What is the book about?

This book shares the inspiring journey of a remarkable child with autism, Nic-Nic— a bright-eyed, curious soul whose world is as vibrant and unique as she is. It invites you to step into her beautiful mind, where dreams dance with imagination, fears coexist with hopes, and every thought reveals a depth of wonder.

Through Nic-Nic's story, you will witness the joys and struggles of a child navigating life with autism, but also the determination of her parents to connect with her. It is a story of love, of hope, and of the relentless pursuit to understand a child whose world operates on its own extraordinary rhythm.

This journey is not only about Nic-Nic's growth but also about the parents and caregivers who walk beside her. It reveals their triumphs and tears, their sleepless nights and small victories, and their unwavering belief in their child. Along the way, it also shines a light on the life-changing work of occupational therapists, who help children like Nic-Nic unlock their potential by easing sensory challenges, building confidence, and empowering their motor and emotional development.

We wrote this book not only for children with autism and their families but also for anyone yearning to understand the beauty, resilience, and complexity of life on the autism spectrum. It is for occupational therapists, teachers, social workers, and anyone devoted to making a difference in the lives of these extraordinary children.

In addition to Nic-Nic's story, this book contains a practical workbook of strategies, techniques, and creative play activities designed to overcome sensory difficulties, improve communication, stabilize moods, and support mental health. These tools are woven with compassion and designed to be used by anyone who wish to nurture a child with autism's growth and happiness.

Above all, this book is a reminder: the smallest acts of kindness—a hug, a gentle word, endless patience, or moments of playful joy—can transform the life of an autistic child.

Thank you for joining Nic-Nic's journey. We hope her story will inspire you, move you, and remind you of the boundless possibilities in every child.

Table of Contents

PART I

NIC-NIC'S STORY

This book tells the extraordinary story of Nic-Nic, a beautiful little girl with autism who sees the world in ways most of us cannot even imagine. Through her story, you'll step into a world where everything is heightened—sounds are louder, lights are brighter, and emotions are bigger. You'll see her hopes, fears, thoughts, and dreams, and discover the incredible ways she longs to connect with her loving parents. Nic-Nic's journey is not just about her challenges and triumphs, but also the unshakable love of her parents and the dedication of passionate occupational therapists who guide her through a world that often feels overwhelming.

Chapter 1
Not A Typical Child

"Autism is a gift wrapped in a mystery." – Keri Bowers

Every child is a universe of their own — a blend of unique abilities, thoughts, and personalities shaped by their environment and experiences. But some children experience the world more intensely, more vividly, and more differently than others. Nic-Nic is one of those children.

I am Angela Maria, an occupational therapist who has worked with children on the autism spectrum. Each one of them has left a lasting impression on me. Maria Shine is an occupational therapist whose niece was recently diagnosed with symptoms related to the autism spectrum.

Both of us created a character Nic-Nic to capture an image of a child with autism.

Every day, Nic-Nic faces a world that is hard to fathom and imagine. The challenges and struggle of Nic-Nic to navigate a world that often misunderstands them fills me with awe. I've seen her hardships in processing sensory and perceptual information, and her progress — the first hesitant steps toward connection, the joyful breakthroughs, and the quiet triumphs.

I've seen the heartbreak of her parents who struggle to understand and reach their child. Parents often come to me with a dream of raising a "typical" child. When they learn their child is different, their world shifts. I've seen the tears in their eyes, their frustration, and the unspoken question: Why my child?

One day, I met Anthony and Aurora, a couple whose lives were about to take a turn they never expected. Anthony was tall, golden-haired, and confident—a successful banker. Aurora was strikingly beautiful, her deep chocolate skin and dark hair reminiscent of a queen. She owned a boutique and salon radiating warmth and confidence. They were extroverts, the life of every party, and together they seemed destined to create a child who would charm the world.

Aurora dreamed of a daughter who would follow in her footsteps. As a former beauty queen, she imagined tea parties, shopping trips, and future pageant crowns. She envisioned a girl who would shine in every room, grow up to be prom queen, and carry her legacy forward.

When Aurora gave birth to Nic-Nic, she thought her dreams had come true. With thick black hair like her mother's and wide gray eyes like her father's, Nic-Nic was perfect. Aurora and Anthony were overjoyed, imagining their daughter as a playful, vibrant child who would light up their lives. But as the months passed, their excitement gave way to confusion, then concern.

Aurora filled Nic-Nic's crib with bright, playful stuffed animals—a giraffe, a dog, an elephant, and a rabbit—expecting her daughter to be captivated. But Nic-Nic didn't respond. She didn't reach for them, or even follow them with her eyes.

At first, Aurora pushed the worry aside. She's just taking her time, she told herself. But more signs emerged. Nic-Nic wouldn't maintain eye contact, even when Aurora cradled her close. She didn't respond to her name or make the cooing sounds most babies make. By nine months, there was still no "mama" or "dada," no gestures, no smiles. The worry persisted.

Aurora and Anthony tried everything to connect with Nic-Nic. They played peek-a-boo. They sang lullabies. They whispered words of love and encouragement. But Nic-Nic remained in

3

her own world, distant and unresponsive. Aurora often found herself staring at her daughter, willing her to look back, to acknowledge her presence. The pain of not being able to reach the child they had prayed so hard for was unbearable.

Yet, even in their sadness, Anthony and Aurora refused to give up. They knew Nic-Nic was special, even if the world couldn't see it yet. They held onto the belief that somewhere inside her quiet world was a spark waiting to be nurtured. They vowed to be her strength, to love her fiercely, and to find a way to help her thrive.

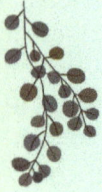

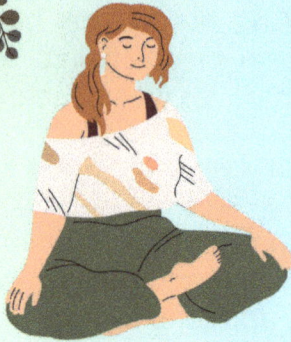

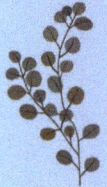

SIGNS THAT YOUR BABY MAY HAVE AUTISM

<u>Sign #1:</u> Very minimal eye contact. Babies should be able to recognize and locate faces by the time they turn two years old. Making eye contact is a way for infants to build relationships with the people around them, especially their parents. But, children with autism don't make eye contact because of social anxiety and sensory overload.

<u>Sign #2:</u> Doesn't babble or point at objects by the time the child turns 1 year old.

<u>Sign #3:</u> Not responding to her name. Most babies respond when they turn 1 year old.

<u>Sign #4:</u> Your baby lacks facial expression. Her face remains blank most of the time. This is because she struggles with social cognition. She can't recognize or interpret social cues.

<u>Sign #5:</u> Your baby doesn't talk much or babble.

<u>Sign #6:</u> Very limited language and social skills.

<u>Sign #7:</u> Doesn't smile or show "happy expressions".

<u>Sign #8:</u> Can't speak short phrases during her first two years.

Chapter 2
A World Of Her Own

Nic-Nic is a child who seems to have stepped out of a fairytale. Her beauty is striking—dark, silky hair frames her delicate face, and her wide gray eyes seem to hold secrets of a world only she can see. She's the kind of child you'd expect to light up a room, but instead, Nic-Nic quietly retreats into a world entirely her own.

While the neighborhood children run and laugh together, playing games in the yard, Nic-Nic prefers solitude. She doesn't join in their laughter or chase after butterflies. Instead, she carefully lines up her toys in perfect rows, absorbed in her meticulous process. To her doting parents, Anthony and Aurora, it's as if their little girl lives behind an invisible wall, unreachable yet full of wonder.

In her quiet way, Nic-Nic paints a picture of autism that is both beautiful and bewildering. Unlike most children, she doesn't look at objects her parents point out to or giggle when they make silly faces. She doesn't clap her hands during peek-a-boo or smile when someone calls her name. Instead, she remains distant, her gaze somewhere beyond the people who love her most. Aurora often watches her daughter with longing, aching for a connection that feels just out of reach.

Despite her angelic face, , Nic-Nic doesn't seek out the company of others. She doesn't enjoy cuddles or the affectionate touch of her parents. While most children run into their parents' arms for comfort, Nic-Nic flinches away, overstimulated by sensations that seem unbearable to her.

Her world is one of rigid routines and obsessive fascinations. She's captivated by toy trains, endlessly enchanted by their spinning wheels, the way they move in perfect lines, and their strict schedules. Hours pass as she memorizes train numbers, engine types, and routes, reciting her newfound knowledge to anyone willing to listen. Trains are her safe space in a chaotic world.

Even the simplest disruptions can throw her into turmoil. If her toys are rearranged, if her daily routine is altered, or if someone takes her favorite spot on the sofa, the result is often a meltdown—intense, uncontrollable, and heartbreaking for her parents. Aurora feels powerless as Nic-Nic cries, screams, and locks herself away. Each tantrum feels like a reminder of how far apart they are, as though they're speaking entirely different languages.

Nic-Nic's hypersensitivity adds another layer to her struggles. Loud sounds cause her to clamp her hands over her ears, wincing in pain. Bright lights feel blinding, certain textures unbearable. Even the smell of someone's perfume or the wrong fabric against her skin can overwhelm her. For Nic-Nic, the world isn't just big—it's too big, too loud, too bright.

Her communication is just as challenging. While other children laugh at jokes or grasp the nuances of sarcasm, Nic-Nic takes everything literally. When her aunt told her to "break a leg," she was horrified, thinking her aunt truly wanted her to harm herself. Phrases like "a piece of cake" left her confused. When someone said that singing was a "piece of cake," she was confused, wondering why anyone would compare singing to dessert. Her speech, too, is unique—emotionless and often in the third person. She struggles to find the right words to express her feelings or needs, leaving her parents guessing and often heartbroken.

For Anthony and Aurora, the disconnect is agonizing. They adore their daughter, but they often feel like strangers in her carefully ordered universe. Aurora watches Nic-Nic spend hours staring at the ceiling or repetitively flapping her hands, and she wants to understand her child's thoughts. "What is she thinking?" Aurora wonders. "What does she need? What is she trying to tell me?"

Nic-Nic's world is a puzzle—a delicate, complex masterpiece that her parents yearn to solve. On some days, they feel helpless, as though they're standing outside a locked door with no key. And yet, even in their frustration, there is love—an overwhelming, unshakable love that keeps them searching for ways to reach their little girl. Aurora dreams of one day finding that missing piece, the one that will let her peek inside Nic-Nic's mind and finally hear her daughter's unspoken words.

Nic-Nic may live in a world of her own, but she is not alone. She is surrounded by parents who adore her, even when they don't fully understand her. And in her quiet, beautiful way, Nic-Nic teaches everyone around her to see the world a little differently—to look beyond the surface, to appreciate the unexpected, and to find beauty in the unique.

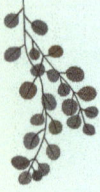

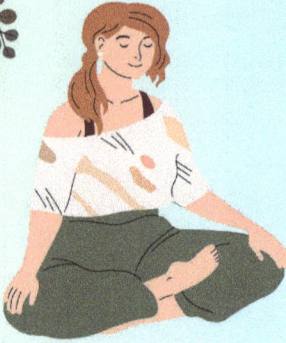

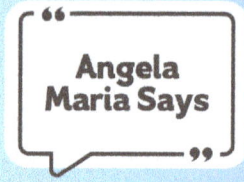

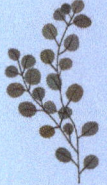

SIGNS THAT YOUR TODDLER OR CHILD HAVE AUTISM

As autistic children navigate the wonderful world of early childhood, they may exhibit the following signs:

Sign #1: They experience social difficulties. They seem to be disinterested in what's going on around them. They show very low interest in establishing social connections and would prefer playing alone. Some of them do not want to be cuddled or touched. Being touched is too much for them. They don't connect with the people around them and they're not very interested in making friends. Sometimes, they ignore people who are talking to them.

Sign #2: They have language difficulties. They use an atypical tone when speaking to others. They often repeat questions rather than directly answering them. They find it challenging to communicate their needs. They do not understand questions, statements and directions. They take things too literally and they don't understand irony or sarcasm.

Sign #3: They also encounter difficulty in non-verbal communication. They avoid eye contact and have difficulty understanding or picking up other people's expressions or tone of voice. They often don't understand non-verbal cues and they often ignore those who try to attract their attention. They are sensitive to loud noises and bright lights. They often have a monotone voice and they have robot-like movements.

Sign #4: They are inflexible. They often have a rigid routine and have difficulty coping with changes in environment or schedule. They sometimes throw a tantrum when their things are rearranged or if their mealtime is slightly different than usual. They tend to repeat specific actions over and over such as rocking, tapping their ears, or flapping their hands. Most of them also like to line up their toys.

Sign #5: They often experience regression. This means that they sometimes lose skills that they have previously acquired. For example, their communication skills or social skills may decline as they age.

Sign #6: Some children with autism are obsessed with certain objects such as toy dinosaurs and toy trains. These s offer a wonderful and unique sensory experience. Everything about trains (their vibrations, colors, sounds, and their organized & lined-up cars) is soothing and stimulating for them. These obsessions are their source of comfort in a world that is too overwhelming for them.

Chapter 3
A Peak Into The Wonderful
But Atypical World Of Nic-Nic

"A World Where Everything's Too Much*

Nic-Nic watches her mom. Though she struggles to read emotions the way other children do, she can sense the heavy feelings hanging in the air—frustration, sadness, and the aching desire to connect. She sees her father sigh deeply when she avoids his eyes, and some days, she watches her mom quietly crying in her room. Nic-Nic wants desperately to explain, to bridge the gap between their world and hers, but the words won't come. So much stays locked inside her, her thoughts swirling like a storm.

What Nic-Nic wishes she could tell her parents is simple: "Everything is louder, brighter, stronger, and bigger in my world. I'm not trying to frustrate you or push you away—I just need you to understand that sometimes, the world is too much."

She wants to say, "I'm sorry, Mom and Dad. I'm sorry for the times I scream, for when I jump up and down or cover my ears. I'm sorry I can't eat something new or try a different route to school. I'm sorry for the tantrums and the tears. It's not because I don't love you. It's because I'm overwhelmed. My world feels like it's spinning too fast, and I don't know how to stop it."

From Nic-Nic's perspective, the world is a kaleidoscope of extremes. The noise of a crowded room is deafening, like a

11

thousand voices shouting at once. Bright lights don't simply shine—they pulse, stab, and dance in her vision. A casual pat on the shoulder feels like a heavy weight pressing down. Even smells, something so small to others, can overwhelm her senses, clinging to her mind and making her feel trapped.

Sometimes, Nic-Nic feels like she's living on a different planet. "People call me a robot," she thinks, "but from where I'm standing, they're the robots—always moving the same way, always understanding each other so easily. I'm not trying to be different. I just... am."

When Nic-Nic is happy, her joy bursts forth. It's not just happiness—it's an explosion of delight, ten times stronger than what others seem to feel. But the same intensity exists for her pain, sadness, and anxiety. Those feelings crash over her like tidal waves, and she has no choice but to react.

She wishes she could explain the meltdowns. "Mom, Dad, I don't scream to upset you. I'm not pulling my hair because I'm angry at you. I'm overwhelmed, and I don't know how else to show it. When my routine changes, or when there's too much noise, I feel like I'm trapped in a room with no doors or windows. It's not that I don't love you—it's that I'm scared, and I don't know how to tell you."

Nic-Nic's struggles stem from sensory processing issues, which make her experience the world in amplified, unfiltered ways. For her, a smell that's barely noticeable to others can be suffocating. A bright light isn't just bright—it's blinding, relentless, impossible to ignore. Even the softest touch can feel overwhelming, like a scratch against her skin.

When a loud sound crashes through her world, Nic-Nic wants to say, "It's not just noise—it's like a thousand drums pounding in my ears. I don't mean to scream or cover my ears to upset you. I just can't handle the sound. It hurts, and I don't know how to make it stop."

Certain smells are equally unbearable. Strong perfumes or fragrant shampoos can make her gag or even throw up. But it's not just bad smells—sometimes even pleasant ones feel like an attack on her senses. The world around her doesn't just exist—it assaults her.

Lights, too, take on a life of their own in Nic-Nic's world. They don't just illuminate—they shimmer, dart, and glare, hurting her eyes and pulling her focus. She can't explain it, but sometimes the light feels alive, almost as if it's chasing her.

She sees the way her mom looks at her during these moments—worried, exasperated, helpless. Nic-Nic wants to reach out and say, "I know it's hard for you, Mom. I know you're doing your best, and I'm not trying to make things harder. It's just that everything in my world feels so big, so loud, so bright. I don't mean to frustrate you—I just need you to understand that this is how my world works."

Deep down, Nic-Nic dreams of a world that feels safe, calm, and manageable. A world where the sounds are softer, the lights are gentler, and the routines stay the same. She doesn't want to disappoint her parents or push them away—she wants them to help her make sense of her overwhelming world.

"Mom, Dad," she thinks, "I need you to be my calm in the chaos. I need you to hold my hand, even when I can't hold yours back. I need you to help me feel like I belong, even when my world feels like it's spinning too fast. Please don't give up on me, because I'm trying—I really am."

Nic-Nic's world is different, yes—but it's also beautiful in its own way. For those who truly listen, who take the time to step into her shoes, her world offers a perspective full of wonder, intensity, and resilience. And in her quiet, profound way, Nic-Nic shows her parents, and anyone willing to learn, that love is bigger than words, bigger than routines, and bigger than differences.

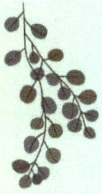

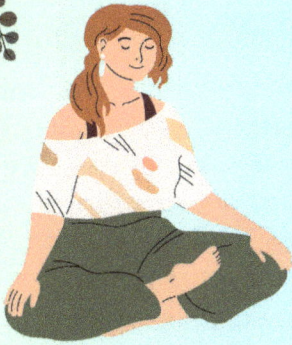

Chapter 3 Notes and Insights

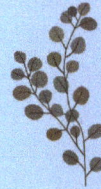

Children with autism see and experience the world differently in a sense that everything seems amplified in the world. Everyday sensor inputs such as light, smell, sound, taste, and touch can be overwhelming for them.

Sight: Children with autism find visual patterns, colors, and shapes overwhelming.

Hearing: Most children on the spectrum are sensitive to unexpected or loud sounds such as sirens, blenders, drills, crying, and car alarms. They are also sensitive to specific or repetitive types of noises such as clapping.

Smell: Some children with autism are sensitive to certain smells, even pleasant ones such as scented shampoos or perfume. Some children on the autism spectrum like to smell everything. Some even notice certain smells that most people don't notice.

Taste: A lot of children with autism like to suck or chew on non-food items such as clothes and toys. They are also sensitive to minty, bitter, and spicy foods.

Touch: Children with autism are sensitive to touch. They are also sensitive to certain textures.

Children with autism often have sensory issues. This means that their brain finds it difficult to take in information from their senses. They have difficulty in processing sensory input such as light, sounds, tastes, touch, and smell.

Though each child with autism is unique, there are **two types of kids in the autism spectrum in terms of sensory processing**. The first type of kids with sensory processing issues are those who are **hyposensitive to input**. Children who are hyposensitive tend to underreact to sensory input. As a result, they may seek more input or more sensory stimulation. This is why they may seem loud, clumsy, or have "attitude or behavior issues".

#1 They are unable to stay still. They have this need to move constantly.

#2 They jump up and down.

#3 Speak louder than the rest of the people in the room.

#4 They stomp their feet when walking, creating loud sounds.

#5 They prefer to play rough when they are in the playground.

#6 They fidget.

#7 They constantly touch other people or objects.

#8 They chew non-edible items such as clothes and toys.

#9 When in class, sensory-seeking kids often won't stop talking.

#10 They often use too much force when drawing. This is why they often break pencils and crayons.

#11 They are messy eaters and often stain their shirts when eating colorful food.

The **second type of kids with sensory issues are those who are sensory-avoiding**. They are hypersensitive to sensory input. Nic-Nic is an example of a sensory-avoiding child. While sensory seekers tend to be loud, children who avoid sensory input appear to be timid. They are picky eaters and they are most likely to:

#1 Dislike being touched, cuddled, or kissed even by their parents or loved ones.

#2 They do not like to wear tight and uncomfortable clothes.

#3 They are sensitive to sound. They can hear background sounds that other people don't hear or notice.

#4 They get startled when there are unexpected loud sounds such as thunder.

#5 They get startled when they're suddenly touched.

#6 They don't like other kids touching them when they're playing.

#7 They have difficulty knowing where their body is in relation to objects and other people.

#8 They don't like being in a huge crowd.

#9 They prefer a quiet environment.

Sensory avoiders, as the name suggests, often avoid sensory inputs such as bright lights and loud sounds because they're overwhelming for them. They also try to avoid being touched or hugged.

Aside from touch, smell, taste, hearing, and sight, there are two other senses that affect children who have sensory issues. The first one is the ability to sense action, movement, and the position of their body in specific space. This is called PROPRIOCEPTION. To put it simply, it is a sense that tells us where our body is in open spaces and in relation to other people and objects. Proprioception is important because it is the foundation of automatic everyday movements. It allows you to take steps without looking on your feet. It is also a sense that we use when we are exploring dark spaces. Children with autism who have sensory avoiding pattern often avoid proprioceptive input. This is why they avoid activities such as riding a horse or a bike. They often hold difficult positions and they have difficulty turning doorknobs or opening doors. They also appear uncoordinated and have difficulty catching balls. They are also experience pain more intensely. They often avoid wearing tight clothing and they often avoid physical activities such as running. They are also overly sensitive to touch and dislikes hugs and other forms of affection.

Autistic children who are sensory seeking or hyposensitive to proprioceptive input, on the other hand, have difficulty avoiding objects when they are moving around. This is why they often crash into furniture and other objects. They stumble and fall often and appear to be clumsy. They have difficulty in maintaining balance. This is why it is hard for them to learn how to ride a bike. They often drop toys and other objects easily. They often try to get more proprioceptive input. This is why they are constantly moving. They jump up and down or flap their hands. They prefer tight clothing and sometimes, they bang their heads on the wall. They also jump or run instead of walking and sometimes, they walk on tiptoes.

The 7th sense that affects children with autism is called the VESTIBULAR sense. This sense affects our movement and balance. Children who are sensitive to vestibular input avoid slides and swings. They are afraid of elevators and they often have motion sickness. Children who are sensory-seeking or hyposensitive to vestibular sensory input love to move and rarely get dizzy. They also love roller coasters and other fast-moving equipment. We will discuss Proprioception and Vestibular Sensory Processing Systems in the next chapters.

One of the things that you should remember is that some children show a combination of sensory-seeking and sensory-avoiding reactions. So, it is important to learn what their triggers are.

Chapter 4
How To See The World
Through Nic-Nic's Eyes

Nic-Nic's world is not like ours. For her, everyday sensations—the rustle of leaves, the hum of a fan, the glint of sunlight—aren't simple background noise; they are overwhelming, all-encompassing forces. This is a child who experiences life tenfold, with every smell sharper, every sound louder, every texture pricklier. Nic-Nic's world is raw, vivid, and relentless.

When her parents, Aurora and Anthony, first brought her to me, they were holding onto both hope and heartache. Their daughter had already been diagnosed with autism, and they wanted answers. Why couldn't Nic-Nic play like other children? Why did she scream at the sound of a passing siren or collapse into tears when routines changed? Aurora's eyes welled with tears as she confessed, "I just want to connect with her. I want her to look at me, to see me the way I see her."

I placed a hand on Aurora's trembling one and said softly, "I know this is painful, but please don't think she doesn't want to connect with you. She does—it's just that the way she processes the world makes even simple gestures, like eye contact, overwhelming. It's not a rejection of your love. It's her way of coping."

The Weight of Eye Contact

Eye contact. To most of us, it's a small, unthinking gesture—a flick of the gaze, a meeting of two persons in shared understanding. But for Nic-Nic, it's a battlefield. Eye contact for her is not just looking into someone's eyes; it's like staring into the sun—too piercing.

I explained to her parents, "In Nic-Nic's world, even meeting someone's gaze is an intense sensory experience. It's not that she doesn't care about you; it's just that maintaining eye contact can feel like being blinded by the sun."

I shared a strategy: "Try to position yourself slightly below her eye level. This makes the experience less intimidating. And when she does glance at you, celebrate it—let her know it matters, not by forcing it, but by gently encouraging it."

Aurora nodded, wiping her tears. Anthony, sitting silently, asked with quiet urgency, "And what about her meltdowns? She screams when there's noise, when we're in crowds, when we're even just a little late. It feels like we're failing her."

Understanding Meltdowns: When the World Becomes Too Much

I took a deep breath, feeling the weight of their struggle. Meltdowns are the language of children like Nic-Nic—a desperate plea for relief when their world becomes unbearable.

"Imagine being trapped in a room where every sound is a scream, every light blinds, and every texture cuts your skin," I began. "That's what Nic-Nic feels in moments of sensory overload. Her meltdowns aren't tantrums; they're her way of saying, 'I'm overwhelmed. I need help.'"

I explained how sensory inputs—bright lights, loud noises, strong smells—hit her harder than we could ever imagine. For Nic-Nic, the sound of a vacuum cleaner is not just loud; it's deafening. The flicker of fluorescent lights isn't just annoying; it's disorienting, as if the world is shaking beneath her feet.

Aurora leaned forward. "So, how do we help her? What can we do when she has a meltdown?"

"First," I said, "don't try to reason with her during a meltdown. She's not in a place to listen. Stay calm, remove her from the overstimulating environment, and ensure she feels safe. Some children respond to hugs during these moments, while others need space. It's important to find what works for her."

I added, "Provide tools to help her cope—things like stress balls, sensory toys, or even noise-canceling headphones. These can act as anchors in a storm."

The Power of Routine in a Chaotic World

Beyond sensory input, I told Aurora and Anthony about another source of Nic-Nic's struggles: change. For children like her, the world is already unpredictable and overwhelming. Routines are their safe harbor, a way to create order in the chaos.

"When you rearrange her toys or change plans suddenly, it's not just an inconvenience for Nic-Nic—it's like her entire world has been turned upside down," I explained.

Anthony nodded, his brow furrowing. "That's why she gets upset even when we're just a few minutes late," he said softly.

"Exactly," I said. "You can help by creating a visual schedule—a chart or series of pictures that show Nic-Nic what to expect each day. This reduces anxiety and helps her feel secure. But life is full of surprises, so it's also important to prepare her for the unexpected. Add a 'question mark' symbol to her schedule to represent potential changes. Over time, this will help her learn to adapt."

Aurora smiled for the first time that day. "You're saying we can teach her to handle change?"

"Yes," I said firmly. "It will take time, but with patience and understanding, Nic-Nic can learn to navigate this unpredictable world."

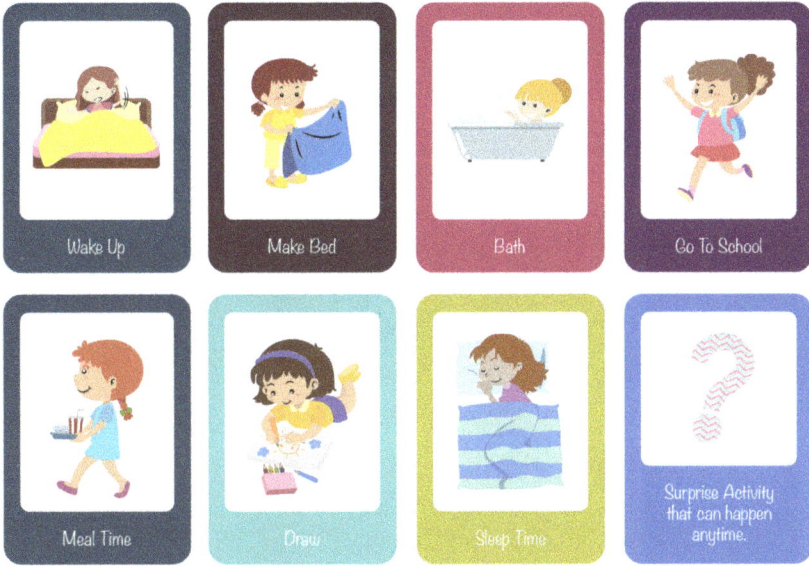

Wake Up | Make Bed | Bath | Go To School

Meal Time | Draw | Sleep Time | Surprise Activity that can happen anytime.

I told Aurora and Anthony that putting a "question mark" in their child's schedule would make it easier for Nic Nic to accept potential changes to her schedule. This will also prevent potential meltdowns in the future.

As I explained everything to Anthony and Aurora, I could see that they were elated. They were beginning to understand the condition of their child and what it takes to help her navigate her world. But there's still so much work to do. Children like Nic-Nic need Occupational Therapists like me who can help them develop skills that they can use for the rest of their lives.

Seeing the World Differently

By the end of our session, something had shifted in Aurora and Anthony. They came to me looking for answers, but what they found was something deeper: an understanding of their daughter's extraordinary world.

Nic-Nic is not broken; she is beautifully, powerfully unique. Her challenges are real, but so are her strengths—her creativity, her honesty, her ability to see beauty in patterns and details most of us overlook.

As they left, Aurora turned to me and said, "For the first time, I feel like we're not fighting against her. We're fighting for her."

And that's the heart of it. Children like Nic-Nic don't need fixing; they need understanding. They need people who are willing to see the world through their eyes, to walk with them through its beauty and its chaos, and to help them find their way.

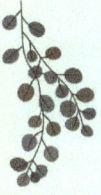

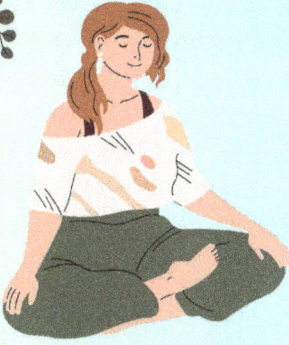

Chapter 4 Notes and Insights

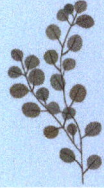

WHAT IS AN AUTISTIC MELTDOWN?

Autistic meltdowns often involve different sets of behaviors such as biting, crying, kicking, yelling, screaming, foot-stomping, and destroying property. Some autistic kids elope or run off while some zone out during a meltdown. Some also engage in self-harm such as hair-pulling or head-banging.

SIGNS BEFORE AN AUTISTIC MELTDOWN

Before a meltdown, children with autism often engage in self-stimulating behavior called "stimming" or repetitive movement. They use this to calm themselves and help regulate their emotions. Stimming actions include finger-flicking, rocking back and forth, hand flapping, watching an object spin (fidget spinner), humming, or repeating phrases.

REASONS BEHIND AUTISTIC MELTDOWNS

Neurotypical kids throw tantrums to get what they want. Children with autism often have meltdowns because of sensory overload. They're overwhelmed. Autistic kids don't act up to manipulate their parents into giving them something that they want. In fact, these meltdowns are caused by stress and anxiety. It is a response to overwhelming sensory experiences. Certain triggers can cause meltdowns such as anger or disappointment. As discussed in the previous chapters, people with autism experience things more intensely. They also feel emotions more intensely. This is why they find it difficult to regulate their emotions. Most kids with autism are not comfortable with social situations so exposure to social events can trigger a meltdown.

HOW TO DEAL WITH AUTISTIC MELTDOWNS AND TANTRUMS

#1 Prevent Triggers

It is necessary that you pay attention and identify your child's triggers. Is it loud noises or unexpected visitors? Ask your child Once you identify your child's trigger, do your best to avoid it or at least manage it. For example, if your child is uncomfortable with having visitors around, you can either avoid having visitors around or tell your child ahead if someone's coming over.

#2 Be Patient

Do not try to discipline your child. Your child is not acting up because he wants to manipulate you. He's having a meltdown because he's anxious and stressed.

#3 Get Rid of the Trigger

If loud music is the trigger, then simply turn it off. You can also use noise-canceling headphones to drown out the noise. If your child is having a meltdown because he's in the middle of a crowd, get him out of there. A noise-cancelling headset can also do wonders for your child.

#4 Give Your Child a Hug

Being hugged is probably one of the best feelings in the world. Give your child a hug when he's having a meltdown. This provides great comfort and security to your child. Remember, do not force a hug. If your child doesn't like it, give him space.

#5 Make Sure That Only One Person Talks to Your Child

Your child is having a meltdown because he's overwhelmed. He will get more overwhelmed if a lot of people are going to try to calm him down. Only one person should talk to your child when he's having a meltdown.

HELP YOUR CHILD DEVELOP COPING STRATEGIES

To prevent future meltdowns, it is important to teach your child coping strategies that he can use to feel calm when exposed to an uncomfortable circumstance.

#1 Teach your child breathing exercises and other muscle relaxation techniques. Train your child to listen to music or take a break when everything seems overwhelming.

#2 Train your child to use sensory aids such as headphones to avoid getting overwhelmed.

#3 When he's stressed, encourage your child to do an activity that he likes such as playing with his pet dog.

#4 Encourage your child to do physical activities such as climbing the stairs, jumping on a trampoline, or doing house chores.

SENSORY AIDS THAT CAN HELP PREVENT ANXIETY, STRESS, AND MELTDOWNS

There are several sensory aids that you can use to help your child manage sensory input and can also regulate his emotions. You can use aids such as sensory (noise-canceling) headphones and your child's favorite perfume. If your child is exposed to an unfavorable smell, spray a little bit of your child's favorite perfume. This will help drown out the unpleasant aroma. You can also use noise-canceling headphones to help block unwanted auditory sensory input. There are a number of other sensory aids that we will discuss later on in this book.

WHAT CAN AN OCCUPATIONAL THERAPIST DO FOR A CHILD WITH AUTISM?

An occupational therapist can help your child manage his condition through the therapeutic use of play and other daily activities. Occupational therapists can help solve the motor and sensory challenges that can hamper the learning and development of an autistic child. Occupational therapists like me can provide therapeutic solutions that target each sense. We provide tools and activities that can help enhance the sensory processing skills of autistic children. We help autistic children improve their daily function and self-care skills.

#1 IMPROVE SENSORY PROCESSING SKILLS

Occupational therapists collaboratively work with parents to help their children cope with sensory overload or overstimulation.

#2 IMPLEMENT DIFFERENT PROGRAMS THAT WILL IMPROVE THEIR DAILY LIVING ABILITIES

Because of sensory challenges, daily living tasks such as brushing teeth or tying shoelaces can be overwhelming for them. Occupational therapists help autistic children perform daily living activities such as bathing, brushing teeth, and dressing.

Occupational therapists create and implement programs that will help your child improve their ability to carry out daily living tasks. One of these programs is to create a sensory circuit that helps energize kids and help them regulate sensory inputs.

A sensory circuit may include activities such as spinning, skipping, and jumping. These activities stimulate autistic kids' central nervous system and will help improve their learning skills. It may also include activities like weight lifting, push-ups, and household chores. These activities can help regulate sensory input.

#3 EQUIP AUTISTIC KIDS WITH EMOTIONAL REGULATION SKILLS

Autistic kids live in a world where everything is intensified. They have intense experiences and emotions. This is why they find it hard to regulate their emotions. Occupational therapists can help these kids improve their emotional regulation skills through role-playing, one-on-one activities and games.

Occupational therapists provide children with holistic and individualized treatment to children with autism. They not only help children with autism improve their motor skills, but their kind and fun demeanor also helps these kids open up to the world and feel accepted and valued despite their condition.

Chapter 5
Nic-Nic And Her Eight Super Senses

Harnessing the Extraordinary Strength of Sensory Integration

Nic-Nic wasn't like other kids, but that didn't make her less—it made her more. From the moment you saw her, you could sense her unique rhythm, a melody composed of quirks, challenges, and hidden brilliance. While other children raced up slides or leapt from swings with ease, Nic-Nic approached the world differently, carefully measuring her every move. She would avoid the swings entirely, overwhelmed by their motion. Yet, at other times, she'd spin in circles, giggling endlessly as though chasing a joy only she could feel.

Nic-Nic's journey wasn't just about navigating the world—it was about rewriting its rules. For her, it wasn't five senses that defined her experience; it was eight.

Unlocking the Mystery of Nic-Nic's World

When I first met Nic-Nic, she seemed like a kaleidoscope—brilliant yet fragmented, colorful but hard to decipher. Her parents, Aurora and Anthony, were at a loss. "She bumps into furniture," Aurora said, her voice tight with worry. "She's afraid of escalators, yet she can't stop climbing on chairs. And her fear of sounds—sometimes even the hum of the fridge—breaks my heart."

Their words painted a picture of a little girl misunderstood by the world around her, a child who experienced life in a raw, unfiltered way that others couldn't comprehend. But to me, Nic-Nic wasn't "broken." She was a puzzle waiting to be put together.

What Nic-Nic's parents didn't know yet was that their daughter's behavior was deeply rooted in her sensory systems. Like all of us, Nic-Nic navigated life through her senses—but hers processed the world in ways that felt overwhelming, disjointed, and at times, magical.

"We don't just have five senses," I explained to Aurora and Anthony. "We have eight sensory systems. And for kids like Nic-Nic, these systems don't always work together seamlessly."

I broke it down for them:

1. *The Basics: The Classic Five Senses*

   - *Sight (Visual)*

   - *Hearing (Auditory)*

   - *Taste (Gustatory)*

   - *Smell (Olfactory)*

   - *Touch (Tactile)*

2. *The Hidden Heroes*

   - *Vestibular System:* This is Nic-Nic's sense of balance and motion. It's why the swings felt terrifying to her but spinning brought her peace.

   - *Proprioception:* Known as the "body awareness" sense, this told Nic-Nic where her limbs were even if her eyes were closed. When she jumped on furniture or crashed into walls, it was her way of seeking—or sometimes losing—this awareness.

- *Interoception:* The least understood of all, this sense helped Nic-Nic recognize what her body was feeling on the inside. Hunger, thirst, and even the need to use the bathroom could feel confusing to her.

The Power of Sensory Integration

I explained to Nic-Nic's parents that sensory integration—the way the brain organizes sensory information—was at the root of her challenges. "For most of us, our brain takes these sensory inputs and blends them effortlessly, like a conductor leading an orchestra. But for Nic-Nic, the conductor sometimes drops the baton."

Aurora's eyes softened with understanding. "So, when she spins in circles or avoids lights, it's her way of trying to make sense of her world?"

"Exactly," I said. "Her actions aren't random. They're a form of communication. And with the right tools, we can help her turn that communication into confidence."

Transforming Challenges into Superpowers

Nic-Nic's behaviors—once sources of frustration—became keys to unlocking her potential. "When she jumps up and down or climbs on furniture," I explained, "it's her way of seeking proprioceptive input. Movement helps her brain organize itself. It's her superpower, not her weakness."

We brainstormed ways to channel this energy productively:

- *Weighted Backpacks or Vests:* To provide the grounding feedback her body craved.

- *Trampolines and Climbing Frames:* Safe spaces for Nic-Nic to explore balance and strength.

- *Fidget Toys and Stress Balls:* Tools to help her focus in moments of overwhelm.

I also introduced the idea of a *"Sensory Corner." "Think of it as her sanctuary," I said, "a place filled with weighted blankets, noise-canceling headphones, lava lamps, and textures she loves. When she feels overwhelmed, this corner will help her reset."

Anthony smiled. "It's like building her own little superhero hideout."

The Magic of Play

Sensory integration wasn't just about tools; it was about connection. Through play, we could help Nic-Nic explore her senses in a way that felt safe and fun.

"Interactive play can change everything," I told them. "It's where NicNic can learn to trust herself and others."

We planned activities tailored to her sensory needs:

- *Blowing Bubbles:* To improve her focus and teach joint attention.

- *Scooter Boards and Animal Walks:* To strengthen her muscles and coordination.

-*Finger Painting and Water Play:* To desensitize her to new textures while sparking creativity.

Each activity was a small step, but together, they formed a path toward independence and joy.

A Sensory Diet Tailored to Nic-Nic

To guide Nic-Nic's progress, I introduced the concept of a **Sensory Diet**—a personalized program designed to balance her sensory input throughout the day.

"Think of it like meal planning," I said. "Except instead of food, we're giving Nic-Nic the sensory stimulation her brain needs to thrive."

The plan included a mix of calming and energizing activities:

- Morning trampoline jumps to start her day with focus.

- Weighted lap pads during meals to keep her grounded.

- Soothing music or white noise to help her wind down at night.

"It's not one-size-fits-all," I reminded them. "As Nic-Nic grows, her sensory needs will change, and her diet will evolve with her."

The Bright Road Ahead

As our session ended, Aurora and Anthony looked at their daughter with new eyes—not as a problem to be solved, but as a story still being written.

"She has so much potential," Aurora said softly, tears glistening in her eyes.

"She does," I agreed. "And with your love and guidance, Nic-Nic will write a story unlike any other—a story of resilience, creativity, and joy."

Nic-Nic may have started her journey in a world that didn't fully understand her, but she was destined to carve out a place for herself, one step, jump, and spin at a time. And as she did, she would teach all of us a little more about what it means to live authentically, boldly, and beautifully.

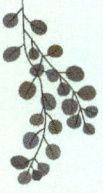

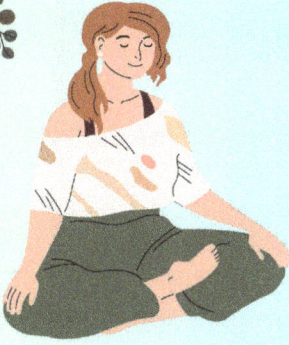

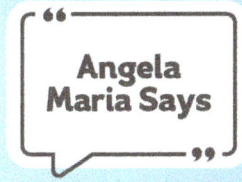

Chapter 5 Notes and Insights

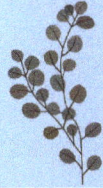

BAD BEHAVIOR OR SENSORY ISSUES?

Because most parents do not have a deep understanding of sensory processing systems, sensory issues are often interpreted as behavioral issues. Children with autism often have proprioceptive difficulties. This makes them challenging or hyperactive. However, some children who have proprioceptive challenges are lethargic and find it hard to cope with social situations. Children with autism jump up and down, they're trying to get more proprioceptive input to give feedback to their proprioceptive and vestibular systems.

TWO TYPES OF SENSORY ISSUES AND PROPRIOCEPTIVE ACTIVITIES THAT CAN HELP REDUCE THESE ISSUES

Sensory issues are divided into two categories- PERCEPTION ISSUES and PRAXIS ISSUES. Perception issues (or Sensory Discrimination Issues) happen when the brain cannot adequately interpret sensory input. Children with perception issues struggle with self-feeding. They miss when they try to put food into their mouth. They also look at their feet when walking or climbing the stairs as they are afraid of missing a step. They find it hard to color inside the lines and they miss the ball when playing soccer or volleyball.

Praxis, on the other hand, is the brain's ability to build a motor plan and execute that plan. Children with praxis issues struggle with movements that are new to them. They have a hard time learning a sport or dance steps. They have poor posture and they find it hard to learn how to write. They also appear clumsy.

There are a several proprioceptive activities that are beneficial to children with autism including animal walks (crab walking, gorilla jumping, frog leaps, bear walks, cheetah runs), jumping, stretching, eating crunchy food, playing catch, and most of all, household chores. Doing household chores can benefit children with special needs because it equips them with life skills that they can use in adulthood. Completing a chore also gives them a strong sense of purpose and accomplishment. It makes them feel good. It also helps them develop empathy.

SENSORY INTEGRATION ACTIVITIES THAT YOU CAN USE TO HELP YOUR CHILD DEAL WITH SENSORY ISSUES

Sensory integration activities are fun play-based activities that help your child deal with sensory issues. Sensory play helps improve your child's creativity, curiosity, problem-solving, and motor skills. These activities help build "nerve connections" in your child's brain making it easier to do activities like walking, crawling, standing on one foot, writing, and drawing. Below are sensory integration activities ideas that you can do with your child:

TACTILE ACTIVITIES	PROPRIOCEPTIVE ACTIVITIES	VESTIBULAR ACTIVITIES
Play in a sandbox	Dance	Balance on one foot

Sensory walk	Climbing the stairs	Sit on a rocking chair
Finger Paint	Lift weights	Play on the swing
Dry Sensory bin treasure hunt	Carry a backpack	Jump rope
Messy sensory bin treasure hunt	Carry grocery bags	Spin ten times and spin in a straight line
Art therapy	Go for a hike	Balance on a scooter board
Sorting activities	Wear arm weights while playing	Jump on a trampoline
Jelly Play	Rake Leaves	Pretent that you are a dolphin & imitate movements of dolphins
Play with water beads	Do yoga	Ride a rocking horse

WHAT TO EXPECT IN THE NEXT CHAPTERS?

The next part of this book is a workbook for parents and children with autism. In the next chapters, you will learn to identify the sensory triggers of your child. You will learn how to create sensory corners and sensory bins. There are self-advocacy strategies that you can teach your child to improve his/her assertiveness and confidence. The next chapters also include affirmations and other tools that you can use to help your child thrive. Lastly, the next part of the book contains self-care strategies that parents can use to make sure that their needs are also met. Remember, you can't pour from an empty cup. You have to take care of yourself, too.

PART II

WORKBOOK FOR PARENTS AND FOR CHILDREN WITH AUTISM

This part of the book contains practical activities, tips, and strategies that parents can use to help their children cope with sensory issues and low self-esteem. In this part of the book, you can find practical tips that you can use to help your child thrive and reach his/her potential. This part also contains self-care and self-love strategies that parents can use to address their own needs. Caring for children with autism is challenging and it is necessary for parents to also take care of their physical and mental health.

Chapter 6
A Place Where Your Child Feels Safe: Creating a Sensory Corner with Your Child

Children with autism live in a world where everything seems too much. Sensory inputs such as lights, smells, sounds, and touch can be overwhelming for them. They get stressed when they feel overwhelmed. Prolonged exposure to undesirable sensory inputs can lead to a meltdown. This is why it is important to create a place where your child can escape whenever he's feeling overwhelmed.

A sensory corner is a place where your child can feel safe. This is a place where your child can feel calm, a place where he can release his fears, anxieties, anger, and frustration. It is a place that can help your child develop his sense and sensory processing systems. A well-built sensory corner increases your child's focus so it's a great place for learning. It also improves your child's sensory processing systems. This means that it can help your child make sense of the world.

IDENTIFY YOUR CHILD'S PREFERENCES

Since a sensory corner is like your child's sanctuary you should fill it with his favorite things. Remember that this sensory corner is for your child so it is important to include him in the process. Take time to ask questions and find out what makes your child feel calm and happy. Then fill his sensory corner with items that can help relieve his stress and frustration.

To identify what your child likes, ask him or her to fill out the following form.

Do you like..?

Angela Maria's Sensory Questionnaire

	Yes, I do.	No, I don't.
1- Do you like it when I hug you?	☐	☐
2- Do you like to squeeze stress balls?	☐	☐
3- Do you like the smell of vanilla?	☐	☐
4- Do you like the smell of pepperment?	☐	☐
5- Do you like to play with paint?	☐	☐
6- Do you like slimy food?	☐	☐
7- Do you like rocking chairs?	☐	☐
8- Do you like colorful lights?	☐	☐
9- Do you like fur?	☐	☐
10- Do you like to play with fidget spinners?	☐	☐
11- Do you like mats that glow in the dark?	☐	☐
12- Do you like lava lamps?	☐	☐
13- Do you like to play on a swing?	☐	☐

ITEMS THAT YOU CAN INCLUDE IN YOUR CHILD'S SENSORY CORNER

Bubble Tube – Bubble tubes are visually stimulating. It has a calming effect.

Mirrors – A mirror can help an autistic child improve his body awareness.

Speakers that play nature sounds – This has a calming effect on your child. But, if your child needs more auditory sensory input, you can play dance music.

Bean bags and cushions – This can provide your child with maximum comfort.

Cocoon Swings – Swinging movement can be therapeutic for kids with autism.

Fidget Toys – These toys can help your child regulate their emotions. They have a calming effect and help improve learning abilities.

TOYS THAT STIMULATE DIFFERENT SENSORY SYSTEMS

PEANUT BALL

This toy helps regulate the senses. Bouncing this ball stimulate your child's vestibular system while rolling the ball over a child with autism can have a calming and grounding effect.

WEIGHTED TOYS

These toys provide proprioceptive input to the joints and muscles and have calming effect. This also enhances focus.

SENSORY BOTTLES

These bottles stimulate your child's visual system. It is also a powerful self-regulation too.

BUBBLES

This has soothing effect. It is also a toll that Occupational Therapists use to help improve the communication skills of kids with autism.

You can also create a sensory corner theme. For example, you can decorate it as a castle or as a forest. Or you can set up a small tent where your child can hang out when he's feeling overwhelmed.

Observe how your child responds to the sensory corner. Remove and add items as necessary. You can also modify the sensory corner later on to cater to the changing sensory needs of your child.

Chapter 7
Proprioceptive and Vestibular Activity Checklist

By now, you already know that the proprioception system is responsible for our sense of body awareness and that that the vestibular system helps maintain our balance. Both systems are important in development, movement, and the ability to carry out tasks.

VESTIBULAR ACTIVITY CHECKLIST

Vestibular activities help improve posture. They're calming and relaxing. They also improve motor skills and help enhance your child's ability to interact with their environment.

Angela Maria's Vestibular Activities Checlist

- [ ] Riding a swing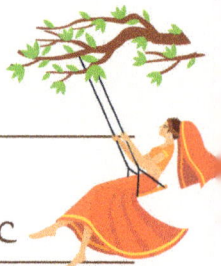

- [ ] Dancing or swaying to music

- [ ] Sitting on a rocking chair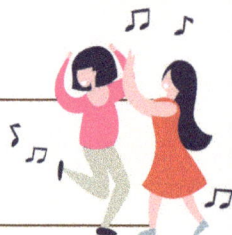

- [ ] Yoga (Inversion Poses)

- [ ] Riding a rocking horse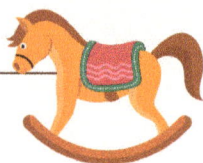

- [ ] Jumping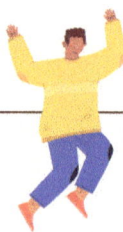

- [ ] Cartwheels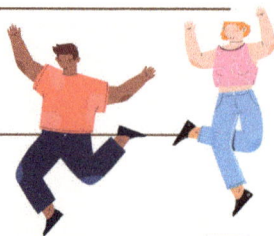

- [ ] Sliding down slides

- [ ] obstacle course

- [ ] Riding a bike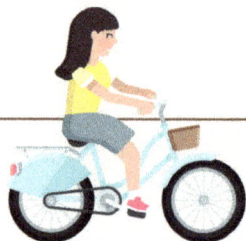

PROPRIOCEPTIVE ACTIVITY IDEAS

Proprioceptive activities have a calming effect. These activities relax the nervous system and improve muscle tone. Doing proprioceptive activities regularly helps improve your child's ability to carry out daily tasks. Below are some ideas that you can use.

Angela Maria's Proprioceptive Activities Ideas

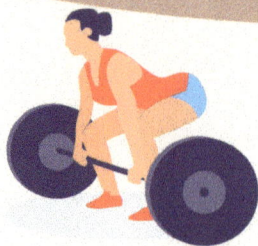

Lifting Weights

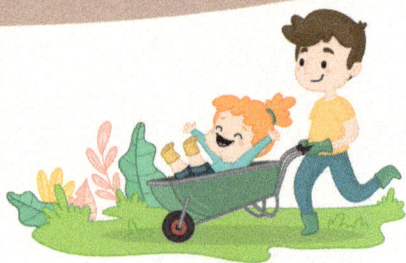

Pushing and pulling a wheelborrow

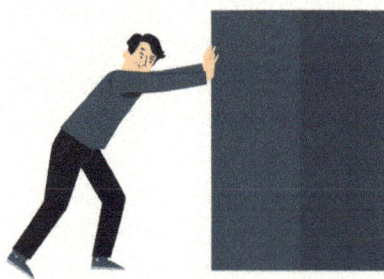

Pushing heavy objects

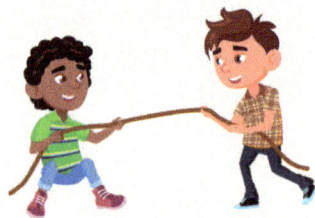

Pulling

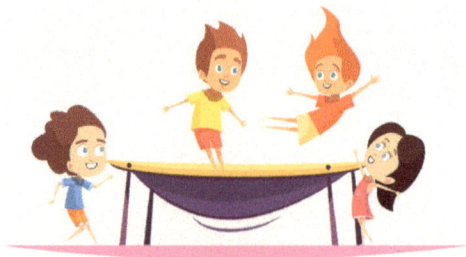

Jumping on the trampoline

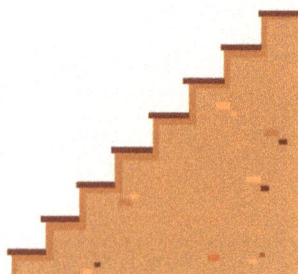

Climb up and down the stairs

ANIMAL WALKS

Animal walks help children with autism develop their gross motor skills. Doing animal walks improves their mobility, coordination, flexibility, creativity, and spatial awareness. Below are some activities that you can try. Try to do vestibular and proprioceptive activities with your child. It would be great exercise for you and it also helps you create a deeper connection with your child.

Animal Walks

FROG JUMPS
hop up and down

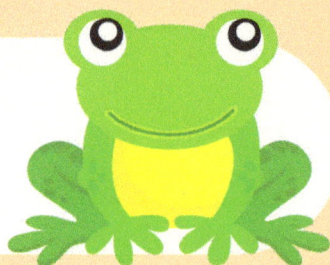

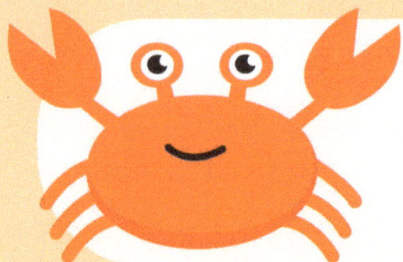

CRAB WALK
put your hands behind you.
Lift your hips and crawl
around just like a crab

CHEETAH RUN
run as fast as you can just like
the cheetah (the fastest animal
in the world). But, you have to
run in place.

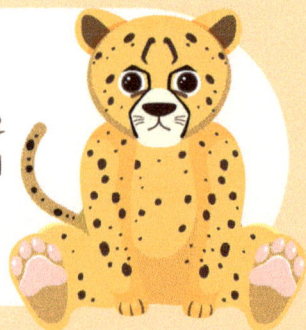

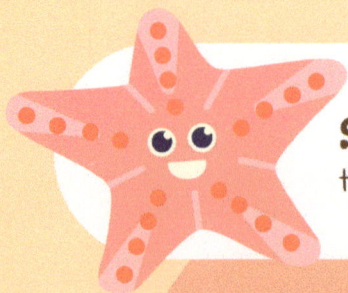

STARFISH JUMPS
this is also known as jumping jacks

Chapter 8
Autism and Assertiveness

Teaching Your Child the Importance of Self-Advocacy

Self-advocacy involves recognizing and effectively communicating one's own desires and needs, as well as standing up for one's rights. By developing self-advocacy and assertiveness skills, individuals with autism - especially as they transition into adulthood - can confidently express themselves, take control of their lives, and make informed decisions. These skills are a hallmark of self-respect and personal empowerment.

However, many individuals with autism struggle to articulate their needs and wants due to feelings of timidity, which can hinder their ability to make independent choices and express their preferences.

To help your child develop these essential skills, consider using the questionnaire in the next page as a teaching tool to foster self-advocacy.

You can also guide your child in developing strategies to handle various situations. For instance, if her friend is playing loud music, you might suggest she say, "Excuse me, I hope you don't mind. Loud music can be a bit much for me since I experience things more intensely than others. Would you be so kind as to lower the volume?"

Encourage your child to share her favorite color and express her feelings by actively listening to her responses. This will help her feel more comfortable expressing her preferences.

A highly effective way to teach your child to assert herself is by modeling self-advocacy. When she observes you confidently standing up for your rights and expressing your needs, it can empower her to do the same.

A key foundation of self-advocacy is self-confidence. In the next chapter, we will explore strategies that can help your child boost her self-confidence and self-esteem.

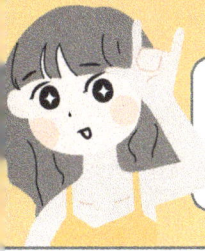

Angela Maria's
SELF ADVOCACY QUESTIONNAIRE

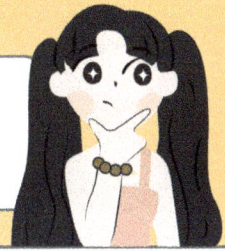

Name:

Preferred Name:

Birthday:

What do you do if your friend's music is too loud?

How do you tell your friend to lower down the volume of his radio?

Describe the most interesting activity you ever did in school.

Do you ask for help whenever you need it?

What is the most important thing you want me to know about you?

Do you tell your family and teachers what you like to do?

Can you describe your weaknesses and strengths?

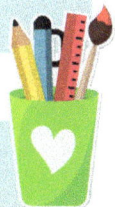

Chapter 9
Strengthening Your Child's Self-Esteem And Self-Confidence Through The Power Of Words

Many children with autism experience low self-esteem due to their awareness of being different from others in terms of interests, social skills, and interactions. They often question why their abilities differ from those of their peers and why they find certain tasks difficult that seem easy for other kids. This can lead to instances where they are excluded from playdates or not invited to parties. Additionally, they may face bullying, as some children may see them as weak or vulnerable.

Moreover, many kids on the spectrum can feel isolated and lonely. They find it challenging to maintain friendships because they interpret the world in a unique way. This sense of being different can make them feel out of place, and despite their efforts, they may find it difficult to accomplish tasks that come more easily to their peers.

How Do You Know If Your Child Has Low Self-Esteem?

Autistic children who have low self-esteem often speak negatively about themselves. They would say things like "I cannot do anything right", "I know that I am different from other kids", and "I am the worst". "Why can't I do this when other people find it easy?", or "I'm stupid". Their negative thoughts are automated. When something happens, they often respond negatively. They are pessimistic. They avoid certain tasks that they find difficult. They don't even try. They have a hard time accepting praise or criticism. They avoid trying new things because they are afraid of making mistakes. They also lack grit. This means that they give up easily when things get hard. Autistic children who have low self-esteem tend to set high expectations for themselves and they aim for perfection.

Individuals with autism who experience low self-esteem often exhibit self-critical behavior. They frequently express negative thoughts about themselves, such as "I never do anything right," "I'm different and I don't fit in," or "I'm a failure." They may also question their abilities, saying things like "Why can't I do this when others make it look easy?" or "I'm stupid." These negative self-statements often become automatic, leading to a pessimistic outlook.

When faced with challenges, autistic children with low self-esteem often respond in a negative manner, avoiding tasks they find difficult and being hesitant to try new things. They may struggle to accept praise or criticism, feeling overwhelmed by the pressure to excel. Their fear of making mistakes leads them to be overly cautious, which can prevent them from developing resilience and grit, as they tend to give up easily when faced with obstacles.

Those with autism who have low self-esteem also frequently set unrealistically high standards for themselves and strive for perfection. This can lead to feelings of inadequacy and reinforce their negative self-image, creating a self-reinforcing cycle that is challenging to break.

What can you do to build your child's self-esteem?

Fostering your child's self-esteem is crucial as it enables them to recognize their unique strengths, personal power, and emotional resilience. Many adults on the autism spectrum struggle with negative self-perceptions and feelings of worthlessness, which can lead them to feel powerless in their relationships. By improving your child's self-esteem, you can provide them with a solid foundation to navigate the challenges they will encounter in adulthood. Here are some strategies you can use to help enhance your child's self-esteem:

#1 Improve your child's self-confidence by highlighting the things he/she is good at.

Many children with autism experience low self-esteem due to a lack of self-confidence. They may perceive themselves as "stupid," "different," or "weak." One effective way to help improve their sense of self-confidence is to highlight their strengths and abilities. Encourage your child to create a list of things they excel at, as shown below.

things
THAT I AM GOOD AT

- Math

- Playing

- Art

- Making new friends

- Drawing

- Science

- Playing the guitar

By Angela Maria

This activity will help children with autism see their worth and value. It helps them focus on the things that they are good at rather than the things that they cannot do.

Always point out the amazing personal qualities that you see in them, things like "You are a fantastic and loyal friend to Cassie" or "You are creative, Nic Nic. Your drawings are amazing". This activity will help children with autism see their value and will help them LIKE and APPRECIATE themselves.

#2 Make a scrapbook containing photos of your child's interests, special talents, and achievements.

This activity will not only help your child develop a positive self-identity. It is also a good bonding activity that you can do with your child.

STRENGTH CARDS

I am good in math	I am a good friend to have	I love to draw and I am good at it
I am caring	I am brave	I am funny
I sing well	What do you usually do in the evening?	How do birds keep their babies safe?

#3 Make a "Strength Card".

Strength cards illustrate your child's strengths or the things that he or she is good at. You can either buy them on Etsy or you can make these cards with your child. You could include strengths such as "I am a great friend," "I am brave,"and "I am kind."

#4 Use the power of positive words.

One of the most effective tools to reduce or eliminate these negative thought patterns is the use of affirmations. But what exactly are affirmations? They are positive phrases or statements that counteract negative or self-sabotaging thoughts. Affirmations can significantly boost confidence and assist children with autism in building resilience and coping with stress. Research published in Social Cognitive and Affective Neuroscience indicates that practicing affirmations activates the "ventromedial prefrontal cortex," a brain region linked to our sense of self-worth (Cascio, N. et al., 2016). Utilizing affirmations for children with autism can enhance their self-worth and self-esteem.

Additionally, it is well-known that children on the autism spectrum often respond positively to reinforcement. This approach not only makes them feel good but also encourages the development of positive behaviors and habits.

SAYING POSITIVE WORDS TO YOUR CHILD

It's understandable to feel frustrated or to use "negative" or "hurtful" language when your child is having a tantrum or behaving in a "difficult" manner. However, using positive words can have a transformative impact on your autistic child. It can boost their self-esteem, foster resilience, and ultimately help them recognize their value in a world that can often be bewildering. Here are some uplifting phrases you can share with your child on a daily basis:

"I love you more than anything in this world."

"I am grateful for you. I am grateful that you are my child."

"You are a gift to us. You are special and I love you just the way you are."

"You bring so much joy into my life."

"You are unique and different in a good way. Know that I love all parts of you. I love you just the way you are."

"You bring love into our home."

"You inspire me every single day. Thank you."

"Your smile brightens all the places you go."

"I believe that you can achieve a lot of wonderful things."

"You inspire the people around you."

"I am proud to be your parent."

"You can do anything you set your mind to."

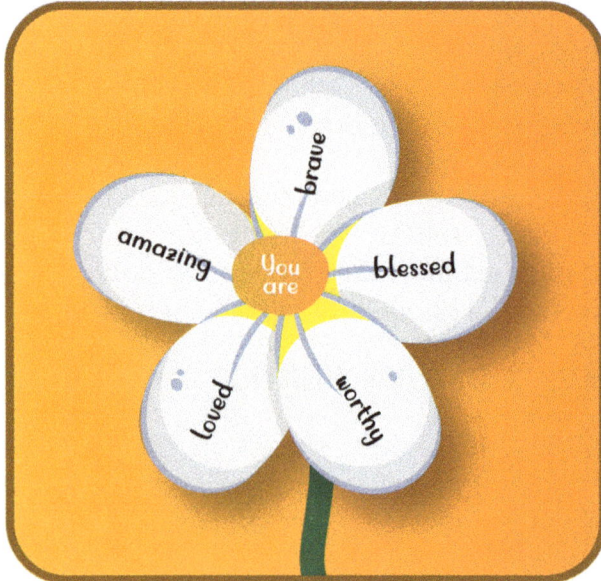

In the next thirty days, tell your child at least one positive thought per day. You can use the following worksheet.

30-DAY AFFIRM YOUR CHILD CHALLENGE

DAY 1	DAY 2	DAY 3	DAY 4	DAY 5
You are enough.	*I am proud of you.*	*You are a gift to me.*	*I love you.*	*I love and appreciate your uniqueness.*

DAY 6	DAY 7	DAY 8	DAY 9	DAY 10
You inspire me.	*Because of you I became a better parent.*	Your smile lights up our house.	*I love that you are unique.*	I accept you just the way you are.

DAY 11	DAY 12	DAY 13	DAY 14	DAY 15
You are awesome.	I'm proud to be your parent.	You are our sunshine.	I love that you are loyal to your friends.	I love that you are good at _____.

DAY 16	DAY 17	DAY 18	DAY 19	DAY 20
Your efforts are appreciated.	You did your best and that's enough.	I love that you are different from others.	You brought so much love into our home.	You are amazing.

DAY 21	DAY 22	DAY 23	DAY 24	DAY 25
You inspire people around you.	You can be who you want to be in this world.	*I love you more than anything in this world.*	Your smile brightens our day.	You bring so much happiness in our life.

DAY 26	DAY 27	DAY 28	DAY 29	DAY 30
I believe in you.	I believe that you can achieve great things.	It's okay.	I appreciate you.	You are valuable.

Use this worksheet for thirty days and see the difference in your child's self-confidence and sense of self-worth.

Using positive language with your child is essential for fostering a nurturing environment that enhances their overall well-being. It helps improve their social skills and facilitates stronger connections and engagement with you. Additionally, it instills a deep sense of belonging and makes them feel cherished.

Affirmation Jar

One effective activity to help boost your child's self-esteem and sense of self-worth is creating an Affirmation Jar. This simple and budget-friendly idea only requires an empty jar, such as a Mason Jar or a used Nutella jar. Begin by writing positive affirmations for your child to read daily. Roll up each affirmation and place them in the jar. Each morning, before your child heads off to school, have them draw a rolled paper from the jar and read it aloud. When they return home from school, encourage them to pick another affirmation to read. Though this may seem like a straightforward activity, it can serve as a powerful tool to enhance your child's confidence and resilience.

AFFIRMATIONS JAR

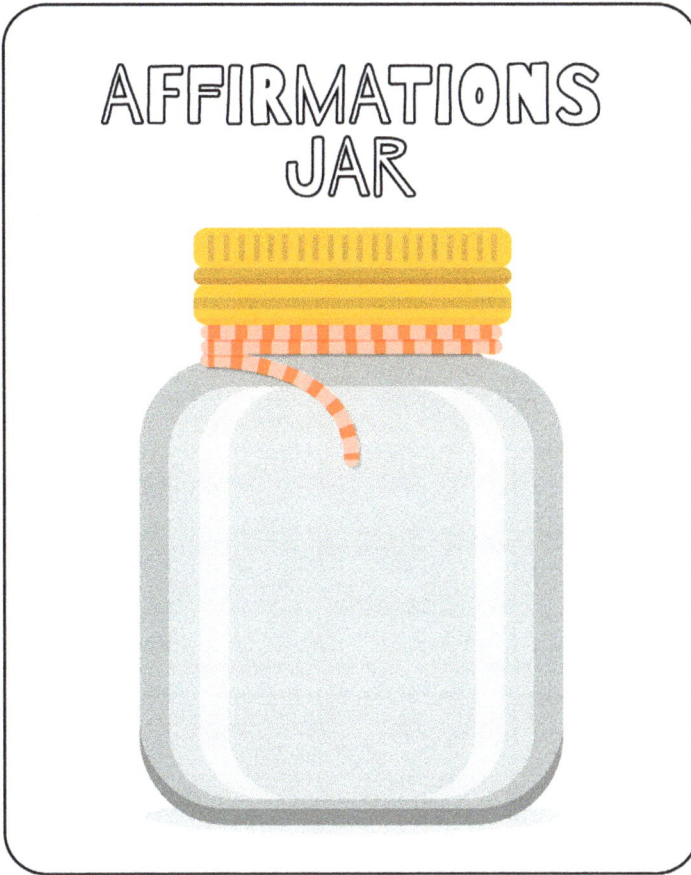

Below are powerful affirmations that you can put inside the jar:

Positive Affirmations for Your Child		
1. I am proud of my self.	16. I am extraordinary.	31. I will do this.
2. I can do this.	17. I love that I am different from others.	32. I can be a super-hero.

3. I believe in myself.	18. I can do hard things.	33. I am good in _____.
4. I am awesome.	19. I am brave.	34. I have a bright future.
5. Today is going to be an amazing day.	20. I am not afraid to try new things.	35. Good things will happen today.
6. I am loved.	21. I deserve love.	34. I am a blessing to the people around me.
7. I am blessed.	22. I deserve kindness.	37. I am not limited by my diagnosis.
8. Being different is a blessing.	23. I can do this and I will do this.	38. I am empathetic.
9. I have amazing skills and talents.	24. I am a wonderful human being.	39. I can make this day a wonderful day.
10. I am good at _____.	25. I am enough.	40. I am capable.
11. I choose to have a good attitude.	26. I do my best and that is enough.	41. I am a good friend to have.
12. I can handle difficult stuff.	27. I am fun.	42. I get better every single day.

13. I am proud of my uniqueness.	28. I see the world differently and that is my superpower.	43. I bring a lot of color into the world.
14. I am different from others and that's okay.	29. I am a wonderful hum	44. I get better and better every single day.
15. I will do great things today.	30. I love myself.	45. I am more than my diagnosis.

Affirmations help calm your child and create a positive environment that is conducive for learning and growth. Positive words help your child regulate his/her emotions and give him/her the strength and confidence needed to face the challenges that he/she will face in adulthood.

Chapter 10
Self-Care Tips For Parents Of Children With Special Needs

Raising a child with autism despite being difficult can be a source of incredibly rewarding experiences. Autistic children often perceive the world in heightened ways, allowing them to feel joy more deeply. They have a unique way with words, creatively describing everyday items—calling ice cubes "water blocks" and electric fans "spinners," for example.

While parenting is inherently challenging, those challenges can be amplified when your child has autism. However, being the parent of an autistic child can also bring immense joy. It strengthens your emotional resilience and reveals the depth of love you are capable of. You might discover a new side of yourself—one that embodies patience and unconditional love. Yet, it's important not to gloss over the difficulties. Parenting an autistic child can also lead to confusion, fatigue, and burnout, making it crucial for you to prioritize self-care. You cannot pour from an empty cup; nurturing yourself is vital so that you can offer love not only to your autistic child but also to your other children and those around you.

Here are some self-care tips to help you maintain balance, prevent burnout, and take care of yourself while supporting your special child:

Tip #1: Have a balanced diet and take time to exercise.

Parents of children with autism often neglect their own nutritional needs and physical fitness. Taking care of a child on the spectrum can be physically taxing. This is why you should take care of yourself and make sure that you have enough energy. Consume 5 to 9 servings of fruits and vegetables, 6 servings of grains, and 3 servings of lean protein. Having enough nutrients will strengthen your immune system. It can also give you the energy and capacity to do your responsibilities as a parent of an autistic child.

It is also best to incorporate physical activities into your daily routine. You don't have to go to the gym every day. You don't have to exercise for two hours a day. Small amounts of physical activity can do wonders for your physical and mental health. It reduces your stress and gives you more energy. It releases a cocktail of feel-good chemicals in your brain such as endorphins. You don't need a gym membership to maintain a regular exercise routine. You can simply incorporate it into your daily life. You can do a 10-minute walk or you can attend a yoga class at least twice a week. This activity grounds you and helps you relax, too.

Tip #2: Build a strong support network.

At times, you feel that you can and should do everything. But it's okay to ask for help. Being the primary caregiver of a child with autism can be exhausting. Thus, it is important to have a strong emotional support group that includes friends, parents, siblings, and other parents who have autistic children. You can also join online communities and Facebook groups where you can learn and share ideas and experiences.

Tip #3: Check available Respite Care Options.

You can also avail of respite care to enable you to rest every now and then. There are many types of respite care including a stay-out caregiver, drop-off programs, and weekly respite programs such as camps and residential facilities.

Tip #4: Make time for yourself.

It can feel like your life revolves around your autistic child, but it's also important to prioritize your own well-being. The ongoing responsibilities of being a parent to a child on the autism spectrum can be physically and emotionally draining, potentially leading to burnout. That's why it's crucial to carve out time to recharge and take care of yourself. You need to make space for your own needs as well.

Make sure to include "me time" in your routine. There are many ways to nurture yourself. For instance, set aside two hours each week for Netflix, or schedule time for a nap or yoga. Treat yourself to a pedicure or massage when needed. You could also enroll in classes that help you learn something new, like accounting, Ikebana, or makeup.

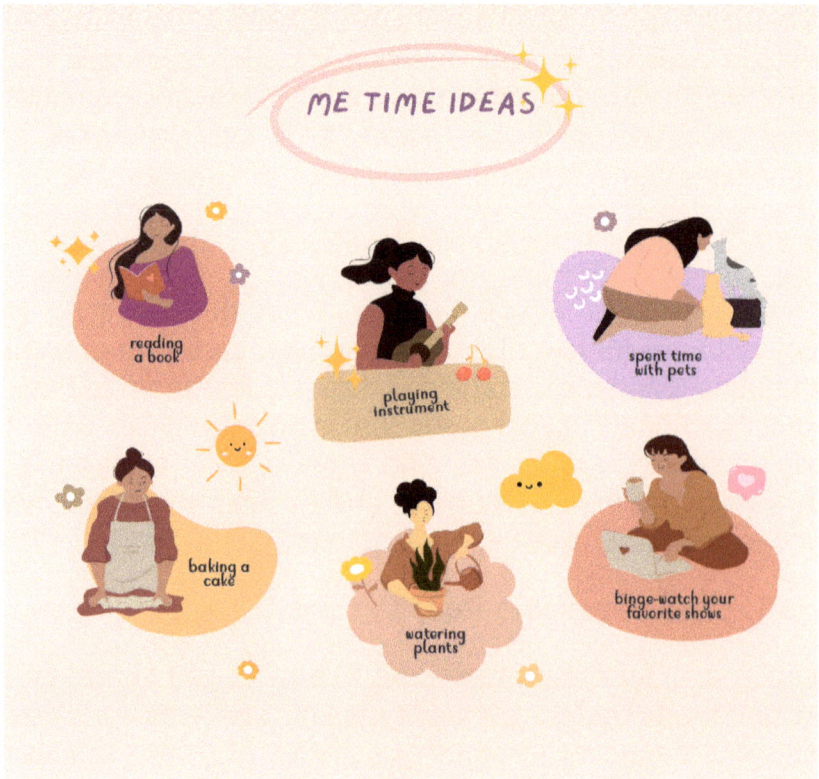

ME TIME IDEAS

reading a book

playing instrument

spent time with pets

baking a cake

watering plants

binge-watch your favorite shows

Tip #5: Take time to socialize.

Your child is precious but he/she doesn't have to be your whole world. You should also take time to socialize and make new friends. See your closest friends when you can. Having meaningful friendships and going to social events once-in-a-while can do wonders in your life. It makes you feel that even if most of your days revolve around your child, you still have a life of your own.

Tip #6: Take Deep Breaths

When everything feels overwhelming, take a moment to pause and focus on deep breathing. This simple act helps manage stress and brings you back to the present, offering relief from anxiety. Even just a few minutes can ease your worries. Dr. Howard LeWine of Harvard University explains that deep breathing triggers a relaxation response in the body.

Tip #7: Be kind to yourself.

There will be days when you feel like what you're doing isn't enough. But remember, you're doing the best you can, and that's perfectly okay. That's enough. There's no need to feel guilty. Practice self-compassion. It's important not to push away negative emotions, as it's natural to feel them. However, try to challenge the voice in your head that tells you you're not good enough or failing as a parent. Be kind and patient with yourself. Speak kindly to yourself. Below are some positive affirmations you can say to yourself each day.

Affirmations for Parents of Children with Special Needs		
1. I am the kind of parent that my child needs.	18. I will be a good role model to my child.	35. I have so much love in my heart.
2. I know that being a parent of a child on the autism spectrum is challenging. But I got this.	19. It is okay to ask for help. I deserve to get hel	36. I try to find love and happiness. I avoid finding faults
3. This, too, shall pass.	Today is going to be a good day for me and my loved ones.	37. I focus on the progress of my child. Not the end result. He/she will get there.
4. I am a good parent.	19. I believe in myself. I got this.	38. I know that my situation is hard. But, I got this.
5. I do my best and that's enough.	22. When I am taking care of myself, I am also teaching my child the value of self-love and self-care.	39. Being a special needs parent is a blessing.
6. I can handle every challenge that life throws at me.	23. I acknowledge the negative things that is happening around me. But, I choose to focus on the positive.	40. I have so much love in my heart.

7. I am my child's most loving and supportive advocate.	24. I choose positivity and optimism.	41. I am doing an amazing job.
8. I am a nurturing mother.	25. I can do this. I can overcome challenges.	42. I am grateful for my child. I appreciate his/her uniqueness.
9. I celebrate the uniqueness of my child. I can see his/her potential.	26. I am enough. I am doing the best that I can.	43. I am resilient and so is my special child.
10. I believe in my child.	27. I am a capable mother.	44. My child is worth every effort and every sleepless night.
11. I believe in myself. I am doing the best that I can.	28. I love and validate myself.	45. I celebrate my progress. I also celebrate my child's progress.
12. I am empowered.	29. I focus on what I can control. I choose to accept and not stress about the things that I cannot change.	46. I choose not to compare the progress of my child to some-one else's. This is just a waste of energy and time.
13.I am learning as I go and that's okay.	30. I accept my child just the way he/she is.	47. I am worthy of respect.

14. My feelings are valid.	31. It's okay to start again. Tomorrow is a new day.	48. My presence is a gift to my child and to the people around me.
15. It's okay to feel tired sometimes.	32. I can get through this.	49. I am proud of the parent that I am becoming.
16. I choose to take care of myself.	33. I am strong.	50. I am a wonderful parent.
17. I forgive myself. I know that I am doing my best.	34. I celebrate good days and I accept that there will be bad days.	51. I am my child's most powerful advo-cate. I will always fight for my child.

WHY IS IT IMPORTANT TO TAKE CARE OF YOURSELF?

As a caregiver to a child with autism, it's easy to become overwhelmed by the endless tasks and responsibilities. There are times when it feels frustrating, and you might even question if you're failing as a parent. But remember, you are doing your best, and that is enough. It's also important to take care of yourself and recognize your own value. You are not just a parent to an autistic child—you are a person, too. Allow yourself breaks, honor your dreams, and fill your heart with self-love. You might think it's impossible to find time for yourself with everything on your plate, but even just five minutes to breathe, engage in something you enjoy, or speak kindly to yourself is more than enough.

CONCLUSION:
A Letter of Gratitude: Embracing the Gift of Autism

Having a child with autism is a profound and life-changing gift. It opens doors to a world you never knew existed—a world that teaches you the depths of your own heart, resilience, and capacity for unconditional love. It is through this journey that you discover a strength within yourself, a strength that allows you to embrace not only your child's uniqueness but also your own.

We hope this book has been a guiding light, helping you step into the extraordinary mind of a child with autism. Our goal has been to offer you practical strategies, compassionate insights, and heartfelt lessons to nurture your child and support their incredible journey. Most importantly, we hope this book has inspired you to celebrate your child's individuality—their clever ideas, vivid imaginations, unique perspectives, and even the behaviors that can seem puzzling at first but are deeply meaningful when understood.

Autism is not a limitation; it is a different lens through which to view the world. It challenges us to rethink conventional ideas of success, joy, and connection. It teaches us to meet our children where they are, to embrace their repetitive behaviors as forms of comfort, to marvel at their creative minds, and to understand their deep need for both independence and safety.

Building a Home of Love and Purpose

We hope this book has helped you create an "autism-friendly home"—a sanctuary where your child feels loved, understood, and supported. A home where differences are not just tolerated but celebrated, where every quirk is seen as part of a beautifully intricate personality, and where your child's voice is heard and valued.

Parenting a child with autism is about more than teaching skills or addressing challenges; it's about fostering a life filled with love, compassion, and purpose. Your unwavering belief in your child's potential is the cornerstone of their growth. With every word of encouragement, every moment of patience, and every step forward, you are shaping a brighter future— not only for your child but for your entire family.

Celebrating Growth Together

As you've explored the pages of this book, we hope you've found joy in the small victories: a new word spoken, a new task completed, or a smile that lights up the room. These moments, though they may seem small to others, are monumental for a child with autism and for the family that loves them.

We've also shared tools and activities to support your child's development—ways to improve motor skills, problem-solving abilities, and sensory processing. But beyond these strategies, the greatest gift you can give your child is the assurance that they are seen, loved, and valued exactly as they are.

A Journey of Transformation

This book is not just about helping your child; it's also about helping *you*—as a parent, a caregiver, and a person. Through the challenges and triumphs of raising a child with autism, you have likely discovered a new perspective on life.

You've learned patience when days felt overwhelming. We hope you've found hope in the smallest signs of progress, and embraced love in its purest, most unconditional form.

Autism transforms families, not by forcing them to "fix" or "change" their child, but by teaching them to see the beauty in the unexpected. It calls on you to set aside preconceived notions and instead focus on the wonder of connection, growth, and shared purpose.

A Heartfelt Thank You

This book is just the beginning of a series, but we want to take a moment to thank you for joining us on this journey. By reading these pages, you've taken a powerful step toward understanding and embracing the unique beauty of autism. Your commitment to learning, loving, and supporting your child is a testament to the incredible parent you are.

Our deepest gratitude goes to you—for your time, for your trust, and for allowing us to be part of your journey. This book was written with the hope of changing lives, and we believe that change begins with you. Together, let's continue to build a world where every child, regardless of their differences, feels cherished and empowered to shine.

With love and appreciation,

Jil and Maria

www.ingramcontent.com/pod-product-compliance
Lightning Source LLC
Chambersburg PA
CBHW052120030426
42335CB00025B/3064